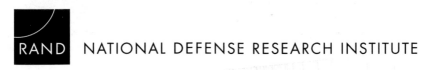

NATIONAL DEFENSE RESEARCH INSTITUTE

T0108781

LIMB SALVAGE AND RECOVERY AFTER SEVERE BLAST INJURY

LITERATURE REVIEW
for the Eighth Department of Defense International State-of-the-Science Meeting on Blast Injury Research

Charles C. Engel, Molly M. Simmons, Sara E. Heins,
Mimi Shen, Gulrez Shah Azhar, Tepring Piquado

Prepared for the Defense Health Agency

Approved for public release; distribution unlimited

For more information on this publication, visit www.rand.org/t/RRA199-1

Library of Congress Cataloging-in-Publication Data is available for this publication.
ISBN: 978-1-9774-0511-1

Published by the RAND Corporation, Santa Monica, Calif.
© Copyright 2020 RAND Corporation
RAND® is a registered trademark.

Cover: photos from DoD, U.S. Navy, U.S. Army, USMC.

Limited Print and Electronic Distribution Rights

This document and trademark(s) contained herein are protected by law. This representation of RAND intellectual property is provided for noncommercial use only. Unauthorized posting of this publication online is prohibited. Permission is given to duplicate this document for personal use only, as long as it is unaltered and complete. Permission is required from RAND to reproduce, or reuse in another form, any of its research documents for commercial use. For information on reprint and linking permissions, please visit www.rand.org/pubs/permissions.

The RAND Corporation is a research organization that develops solutions to public policy challenges to help make communities throughout the world safer and more secure, healthier and more prosperous. RAND is nonprofit, nonpartisan, and committed to the public interest.

RAND's publications do not necessarily reflect the opinions of its research clients and sponsors.

Support RAND
Make a tax-deductible charitable contribution at
www.rand.org/giving/contribute

www.rand.org

Preface

This report was intended to facilitate the Eighth Department of Defense (DoD) International State-of-the-Science Meeting (SoSM) on Blast Injury Research. The SoSM series was established in 2009 under the authority of the DoD Executive Agent (EA) for Blast Injury Research. Its purpose has been to identify knowledge gaps in blast injury research; ensure that DoD medical research programs address existing gaps; foster collaboration between scientists, clinicians, and engineers in blast injury–related fields; promote information sharing on the latest research; and identify immediate, short-term, and long-term actions to prevent, mitigate, and treat blast injuries. The eighth SoSM topic was "Limb Salvage and Recovery After Blast-Related Injury."

A foundational part of each SoSM consensus process is a comprehensive background literature review. This review provides an overview of the literature and delivers a series of recommendations for future medical research relating to limb salvage, emphasizing prevention, mitigation, and treatment research and recommendations. This work may be of interest to senior military and medical leaders, DoD policymakers, military and veterans research portfolio managers, and healthy and injured military service members and their families.

This research was sponsored by the the DoD Blast Injury Research Coordinating Office and conducted within the Forces and Resources Policy Center of the RAND Corporation's National Defense Research Institute, a federally funded research and development center sponsored by the Office of the Secretary of Defense, the Joint Staff, the Unified Combatant Commands, the Navy, the Marine Corps, the defense agencies, and the defense intelligence enterprise.

For more information on the RAND Forces and Resources Policy Center, see www.rand.org/nsrd/frp or contact the director (contact information is provided on the webpage).

Contents

Figure and Tables

Figure

Tables

Summary

Introduction

The conflicts in Iraq and Afghanistan have led to important changes in the mechanism, severity, and complexity of blast-related battlefield injuries, largely because of the advent and increased enemy-combatant use of improvised explosive devices. These changes have led to more-frequent blast-related traumatic injuries among deployed service members. However, because of military medical advances and improvements in protective equipment, a greater proportion of blast-exposed service members are surviving despite their severe injuries. Also, advances in surgical reconstruction and rehabilitation have led to an increased medical capacity to salvage limbs that, until recently, would have resulted in amputation. Collectively, these developments have led to important questions about when and how to emphasize limb salvage over amputation after severe blast-related limb injuries.

The U.S. Department of Defense (DoD) Blast Injury Research Coordinating Office (BIRCO) sponsored the Eighth Department of Defense International State-of-the-Science Meeting (SoSM) on Blast Injury Research to identify what is known and not known (knowledge gaps) pertaining to key blast injury–related topics and emerging issues. The topic of the SoSM was "Limb Salvage and Recovery After Severe Blast Injury." To inform the SoSM and the associated consensus process, the BIRCO requested that the RAND Corporation's National Defense Research Institute conduct a comprehensive literature review on limb salvage following severe blast injury. For the purposes of this review and in consultation with the SoSM planning committee members (see the appendix), *blast-related limb salvage* is described as the restoration of limb and individual to maximum function after severe blast-related limb injury.

We also developed four main literature review objectives:

1. Describe the epidemiology and outcomes of limb salvage after severe blast-related limb injury.
2. Review the evidence about the decision to salvage versus amputate a limb after severe blast-related limb injury.
3. Examine evidence and innovations about restoration and reconstruction after limb salvage for severe blast-related limb injury.
4. Review evidence and innovations about rehabilitation, reintegration, and recovery after limb salvage for severe blast-related limb injury.

We sought to review studies to help us better understand blast-related limb salvage, particularly as the research pertained to our four objectives. This search yielded 184 articles that met final full text review and 105 articles that met final inclusion criteria.

Findings and Recommendations

In presenting the findings from those 105 articles, we broke the literature into epidemiologic, basic, and clinical research. Details on these findings can be found in the report, but the overall finding is that there is a very limited body of empirical research on blast-related injuries to extremities and subsequent limb salvage; much more research is needed. To focus our review findings and recommendations, we used the four literature review objectives as an organizational structure.

Describe the Epidemiology and Outcomes of Limb Salvage After Severe Blast-Related Limb Injury

Findings

Severe limb injuries are common among combat-injured service members. Persistent and disabling pain, sleep disturbance, depression and anxiety, and general loss of functioning are common after these injuries. Most service members with severe combat-related limb injury are significantly disabled. An important gap is the absence of completed prospective, longitudinal studies with follow-up longer than one year.

Recommendations

We recommend establishing theater-wide medical surveillance systems (e.g., Military Orthopaedic Trauma Registry), coupled with studies with follow-up of more than one year with military and U.S. Department of Veterans Affairs collaboration. This will facilitate research to validate outcome measures, estimate rates of complications, improve prognostication methods, identify optimal candidates for limb-salvage efforts, and initiate prospective, longitudinal cohort studies with long follow-up. Presently, because the casualty flow is low, DoD extremity trauma research cannot be meaningfully conducted. Thus, we also recommend that DoD establish and maintain relationships with civilian trauma centers and research platforms to support further research.

Review the Evidence About the Decision to Salvage Versus Amputate a Limb After Severe Blast-Related Limb Injury

Findings

To date, prognostic assessment tools have largely failed as decision aids for clinicians and patients. There is no one-size-fits-all intervention for severe blast-related limb injuries, and there is a need for ongoing, intensive efforts to share and study decisionmaking with patients, caregivers (as appropriate), and a multidisciplinary clinical team. Furthermore, there is limited evidence on the outcomes of amputation versus limb salvage overall and in clinically relevant subgroups.

Recommendations

We recommend that, during peace, longitudinal studies and controlled clinical trials that address decisionmaking and clarify the relative merits of limb salvage versus amputation should recruit patients from the vast U.S. network of civilian trauma centers. We further recommend that future research explore feasible clinical models of shared decisionmaking, patient-centered treatment planning, and patient-reported outcomes pertaining to limb salvage–related decisions following severe limb trauma. We recommend that military hospitals partner with civilian trauma centers and extremity trauma research platforms investigate the impact of military clinician training in such settings on the development and maintenance of limb salvage–related skills among military clinicians and to strengthen research ties.

Examine Evidence and Innovations About Restoration and Reconstruction After Limb Salvage for Severe Blast-Related Limb Injury
Findings

Current evidence comparing various surgical approaches to limb salvage for blast-related limb injury is preliminary at best.

Recommendations

As new salvage techniques are introduced, we recommend that a series of large, multicenter trials enrolling civilians is instituted. Depending on the military tempo of combat operations occurring in parallel with these studies, it might be possible to include patients with high-energy sources of severe limb injuries from both military and civilian populations. This multicenter approach will maximize the likelihood of enrolling enough patients to obtain adequate statistical power to identify clinically important differences in outcomes when comparing treatment strategies.

Review Evidence and Innovations About Rehabilitation, Reintegration, and Recovery After Limb Salvage for Severe Blast-Related Limb Injury
Findings

The most underdeveloped area of empirical research we reviewed pertained to rehabilitative approaches in caring for blast-injured patients with severe limb injuries. Promising programs have been identified, but codification and empirical evaluation are needed.

Recommendations

We recommend research into complex multidisciplinary rehabilitation and reintegration strategies to support service members and their caregivers in achieving recovery and possibly a return to military service. We recommend codifying complex rehabilitative interventions for limb-salvage patients and further exploring the feasibility, important outcomes, assessments of intervention fidelity, and specific randomized designs that are most appropriate for studying the effectiveness of complex rehabilitative strategies for blast-related limb salvage and recovery. Again, it might be possible to include patients with high-energy sources of severe limb injuries from both military and civilian populations. We also recommend developing validated outcome measures on limb strength, performance, and function, as well as rehabilitative psychosocial interventions that reduce service members' suffering from chronic pain, persistent sleep disorders, posttraumatic stress disorder (PTSD), anxiety, and related consequences of these injuries. Finally, the signature orthopedic advance from the Operation Iraqi Freedom and Operation Enduring Freedom conflicts might be developing, perfecting, and deploying the dynamic ankle-foot orthosis in caring for severe lower-extremity injuries. This area needs continued focus, with an emphasis on continued improvement and broader application.

Acknowledgments

We gratefully acknowledge Michael Leggieri, Raj Gupta, and COL Sidney Hinds of BIRCO for their comments, guidance, and support of this project. We also wish to recognize the extensive work that BIRCO has done prior to RAND involvement, refining DoD's State-of-the-Science Meeting process from which this literature review has emerged, a process that BIRCO has used to develop DoD research policy and priorities related to blast injury since 2009.

We are indebted to all of those whom we consulted regarding topic selection, as well as the State-of-the-Science Meeting planning committee and expert panel. These individuals provided us with invaluable guidance for the preparation of this literature review and for virtually all other aspects of this eighth meeting in the ongoing series of international DoD State-of-the-Science Meetings on Blast Injury Research.

We extend special thanks to Samantha McBirney and Stephanie Holliday for their assistance in reviewing and editing the manuscript, Jody Larkin and Elizabeth Hammes for their help with the literature search, Paul Steinberg and Emily Ward for their careful edits, Lee Remi and Sale Lilly for their work and project assistance, and Craig Bond, Saci Detamore, and Tracey Cook for their assistance with project management and quality assurance.

Abbreviations

AFO	ankle-foot orthosis
BIRCO	Blast Injury Research Coordinating Office
CTA	computed tomographic angiography
DoD	U.S. Department of Defense
DTIC	Defense Technical Information Center
FIM	Functional Independence Measure
HiMAT	High-Level Mobility Assessment Tool
IED	improvised explosive device
LEAP	Lower Extremity Assessment Project
LEFS	Lower Extremity Functional Scale
MCS	Mental Component Score
MESS	Mangled Extremity Severity Score
METALS	Military Extremity Trauma Amputation/Limb Salvage
METRC	Major Extremity Trauma Research Consortium
PTSD	posttraumatic stress disorder
RTR	Return to Run
SF-12	Short-Form 12 item
SIP	Sickness Impact Profile
SMFA	Short Musculoskeletal Function Assessment
SoSM	State-of-the-Science Meeting
VA	U.S. Department of Veterans Affairs

VAVIS   U.S. Department of Veterans Affairs Vascular Injury
               Study
VST   virtual stress testing

CHAPTER ONE

Background and Purpose

Background

During the conflicts in Iraq and Afghanistan, there have been important changes in the mechanism, severity, and complexity of blast-related battlefield injuries, largely because of the advent and increased enemy combatant use of improvised explosive devices (IEDs). Although explosive blast in the theater of combat operations is not new, the rise in IEDs has changed the nature of extremity injuries from what it was in previous conflicts. The result has been more-frequent blast-related physical injuries among deployed service members and the more-regular need for acute medical responses directed toward the life-threatening complications associated with these injuries. Blast exposures create wide bone and tissue injury not seen in other types of extremity injuries. Furthermore, blast-related bone injuries might not result in the types of fractures that orthopedic surgeons are accustomed to regularly seeing (Keeling et al., 2010; Owens et al., 2007).

Hidden explosives, such as IEDs, landmines, and booby traps, are to blame for as much as half of the injuries seen in field hospitals (Ramasamy et al., 2009). Most of these injuries are to lower extremities (Balazs et al., 2014). Military medical advances and improvements in protective equipment have resulted in greater survival despite severe blast-related injuries, and advances in surgical reconstruction and rehabilitation have resulted in an increased medical capacity to salvage limbs that previously would have been amputated. Collectively, these developments have led to important questions about when and how to emphasize limb salvage after severe blast-related limb injuries.

The U.S. Department of Defense (DoD) Blast Injury Research Coordinating Office (BIRCO) sponsored the Eighth Department of Defense International State-of-the-Science Meeting (SoSM) on Blast Injury Research. The goal of the SoSM and associated processes is to identify what is known and not known (knowledge gaps) about key blast injury–related topics and emerging issues. The topic of the SoSM was "Limb Salvage and Recovery after Severe Blast Injury."

Purpose of the Review

To inform the SoSM and the associated consensus process, the BIRCO requested a comprehensive literature review on limb salvage following severe blast injury. This review focuses on scientific evidence from the academic and gray literature. For this review, the RAND Corporation— with assistance from the planning committee—developed four main literature review objectives:

1. Describe the epidemiology and outcomes of limb salvage after severe blast-related limb injury.
2. Review the evidence about the decision to salvage versus amputate a limb after severe blast-related limb injury.
3. Examine evidence and innovations about restoration and reconstruction after limb salvage for severe blast-related limb injury.
4. Review evidence and innovations about rehabilitation, reintegration, and recovery after limb salvage for severe blast-related limb injury.

Defining Blast-Related Terms

Before proceeding to the literature review, the planning committee, in collaboration with us, discussed the terms *blast-related* and *blast-related limb salvage*, which are used in the review.

The planning committee described *blast-related* as injury from one or more blast-injury mechanisms, ranging from primary to quinary (Department of Defense Directive 6025.21E, 2018). Primary blast injuries involve tissue damage that occurs in response to the direct physical effects of blast overpressure wave. Secondary blast injuries are those produced by fragments from the exploding device or secondary projectiles from the environment (e.g., debris, vehicle fragments). Tertiary blast injuries result from blast-related displacement of body parts that strike other objects, causing a variety of injury types (e.g., blunt, avulsion, crush). Quaternary and quinary injuries result from other explosive products or the clinical consequences of environmental contaminants (e.g., biologicals, radiation, released fuels), respectively. This review, therefore, was concerned with all of these blast mechanisms.

To ensure an expansive search of the literature, the planning committee described *blast-related limb salvage* as the restoration of limb and individual to maximum function after severe blast-related limb injury. There was agreement among the planning committee members that military personnel are a young, active group with higher levels of pre-injury fitness, which places high demands on their postoperative rehabilitation to ensure recovery to previous functional capability. It is also important to note the varied use of the term *limb salvage* in the literature that we reviewed. Specifically, many articles do not explicitly define *limb salvage*; instead, authors refer to it as "not an amputation," "limb restoration," or "limb-sparing" or use these terms interchangeably (Akula et al., 2011; Barla et al., 2017; Bennett, et al., 2018; Blair et al., 2016; Bosse et al., 2002; MacKenzie et al., 2007; Melcer et al., 2017; Owens, et al., 2011; van der Merwe et al., 2016). Limb salvage is also described in terms of procedures, such as involving either local or free muscle flaps or microvascular free tissue transfer for wound coverage, management of vascular injuries, operative treatment and revascularization, bone-grafting or bone transport, repair of a major nerve injury, treatment of a complete compartment injury or compartment syndrome, and plastic surgical techniques (Aoki, 2018; Brown et al., 2011; Chung et al., 2009; Doukas et al., 2013; Penn-Barwell et al., 2015).

The planning committee broadly defined *limb salvage* as restoration of limb, with the goal to include literature that describes new approaches, promising advances of surgical techniques, or improvements in responses following the injury. Additionally, the planning committee suggested this definition and expanded the scope of the search to provide meeting participants with information that might lead to innovative solutions to recovery after blast-related injury.

Organization of This Report

In Chapter Two, we discuss the methodology underlying the literature review. In Chapter Three, we present the findings in terms of epidemiological, basic, and clinical research. In Chapter Four, we discuss the findings in terms of the four literature review objectives and provide some recommendations based on those findings. Finally, in the appendix, we present a list of the members of the eighth SoSM planning committee.

CHAPTER TWO

Review Methodology

We consulted with the planning committee—a multidisciplinary group of experts on blast-related limb salvage and recovery—to develop initial search terms. After agreeing on search terms, we searched the peer-reviewed and gray literature that described the occurrence and treatment of military blast-related limb salvage. Specifically, we searched the peer-reviewed scientific literature on PubMed, Web of Science, and PsycINFO and searched the DoD gray literature on the Defense Technical Information Center (DTIC). The period of interest was calendar year 2008 through calendar year 2018. Additional references were identified that (1) were published prior to 2008 *or* (2) did not meet inclusion criteria but either represented a seminal article (e.g., the original article describing the Parkland Formula for fluid resuscitation among burn patients [Scheulen and Munster, 1982]) or provided context for interpreting the literature.

To initially develop search terms, we provided potential search terms based on the selected topic: blast-related burn injury. Sources included previous literature reviews for blast-injury research SoSMs, terms specifically relevant to blast-related limb salvage and recovery, and associated structured vocabulary (e.g., as listed in Medline Medical Subject Headings [MeSH]) used to search the literature databases noted in the previous paragraph. A preliminary literature search was then performed, and the results were used to improve the initial search strategy. Search terms used are summarized in Table 2.1 in terms of three domains: exposure, population and context, and specific programs.

The literature review included any research that addressed one or more blast-related limb injury mechanisms, ranging from primary to quinary (as discussed in Chapter One), and research that addressed any part of the translational health research continuum, from foundational research to health services research, as defined in the National Research Action Plan (NRAP).

Table 2.1
Search Terms by Domain

Domain 1: Exposure	Domain 2: Population and Context	Domain 3: Specific Programs
blast	limb salvage	Lower Extremity Assessment Project (LEAP)
explos*, explod*	extremity salvage	Outcomes Following Severe Distal Tibia, Ankle and/or Foot Trauma: Comparison of Limb Salvage Versus Transtibial Amputation Protocol (OUTLET)
IED, IEDs	mangled limb	Military Extremity Trauma Amputation/Limb Salvage (METALS)
pressure wave	mangled extremity	Major Extremity Trauma Research Consortium (METRC)
overpressur*	IIIB tibia fracture	
pressure differential	IIIC tibia fracture	
grenade*	extremity trauma	
bomb*	limb reconstruct*	
landmine	extremity reconstruct*	
implosion, implode, imploding	limb recovery	
mortar	extremity recovery	
mine field	limb injury	
	limb trauma	
	extremity trauma	

NOTE: * indicates a variety of words that include a given stem; for example, *explos** refers to *explosion, explosions, explosive,* and so on.

Two trained reviewers performed an initial screen of all citation titles and abstracts from the initial search, and articles were excluded if they were unrelated to the major review objectives (Table 2.2). Only English-language articles approved for general public release were considered. Reviewers compared assessments of inclusion and exclusion criteria to achieve inter-rater reliability and discussed any discordant results between themselves. If discordance was unresolved after their discussion, the review team was consulted to determine the appropriate coding.

For all citations that remained after the initial title and abstract screening, full-text articles were pulled and reviewed. We excluded studies that (1) did not indicate a blast injury or blast assessment; (2) did not involve limb salvage or recovery after limb salvage (most often because all patients received amputations); (3) were an annual report of grant-funded work; or (4) were a commentary or editorial. Subsequent studies were identified based on searches of reference lists, clinical and safety guidelines, policy documents, other relevant gray literature, and planning committee recommendations.

The search yielded 173 unique citations and 11 additional citations identified from secondary searches of reference lists from full-text articles, for a total of 184 citations (Figure 2.1). Given the limited-number of articles, we opted to do a full screening of every manuscript identified. After full text review, 105 of these articles met the criteria for inclusion in the literature review.

Table 2.2
Literature Review Eligibility Criteria

Inclusion Criteria	Exclusion Criteria
English-language articles only	Article did not address review objectives
Adults only	Cancer-related limb salvage
Articles published from 2008 through 2018, inclusive[a]	Commentary or editorial
Human and animal model studies	Administrative protocol or report
Approved for public release, distribution unlimited	

[a] Older publications were included as necessary for background or to address a review objective.

Figure 2.1
Literature Search Flow Diagram

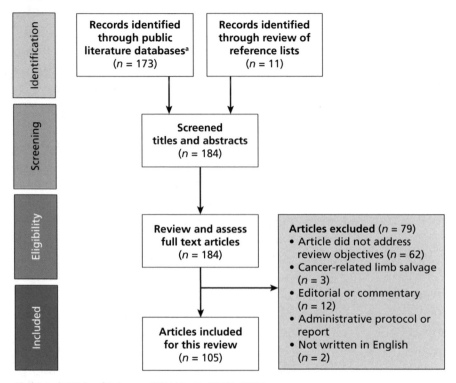

ªPubMed, Web of Science, CINAHL, PsyINFO, DTIC.

CHAPTER THREE

Results

This chapter summarizes findings from the articles meeting our criteria for eligibility. We broke the literature into epidemiological, basic, and clinical research.

Epidemiological Research

Epidemiological studies help characterize the magnitude of the blast-related limb salvage and recovery challenge for the military and common outcomes associated with severe blast-related limb injuries.

A few studies have characterized blast-related injuries, including limb trauma during the armed conflicts in Iraq and Afghanistan. As noted, hidden explosives—such as IEDs, landmines, and booby traps—are to blame for as much as half of the injuries seen in field hospitals (Ramasamy et al., 2009), with the majority of these injuries to lower extremities (Balazs et al., 2014). Research from the United Kingdom showed that, among military personnel, 77 percent of people who were injured while deployed had an extremity injury and 11 percent had at least one amputation. Thirty-three percent of individuals had an upper-extremity fracture, and 67 percent had a lower-extremity fracture. Of those, 69 percent of upper-extremity fractures and 58 percent of lower-extremity fractures were open. This meant that extremity injuries accounted for a vast majority of combat injuries in the United Kingdom (Chandler et al., 2017). However, this research was not specific to blast-related extremity injuries.

Symptoms and functional impairment after severe blast-related limb injury are generally significant, even after substantial periods of rehabilitation. One study of 130 service members with combat-related extremity trauma who were evacuated to Brooke Army Medical Center assessed pain, sleep disturbance, depression, and anxiety using validated measures at the time of hospital discharge. Among those symptomatic patients, 88 percent met study criteria for significant levels of pain, sleep disturbance, depression, or anxiety; physical functioning and mental health functioning were roughly one and two standard deviations below population norms, respectively (Young-McCaughan et al., 2017). In a case series analysis of individuals injured during recent military conflicts who had undergone late amputation following limb salvage, poor mental health and dissatisfaction with limb reconstruction each were cited as reasons for undergoing late amputation in the majority of patients (Krueger et al., 2015).

Basic Research

Our search identified several animal studies addressing questions related to limb salvage. Spear et al., 2015, showed that the endothelium is activated when tissue from rabbit hind limbs is exposed to a blast overpressure in the lab. The authors attempted to link the findings to poor limb-salvage outcomes, suggesting that this endothelial activation might cause pathological changes in the surrounding tissues. Shaw et al., 2017, investigated the impact of blast overpressure exposure on cartilage in the hind legs of pigs. The researchers found that evidence of increased chondrocyte death in the cartilage of these limbs was associated with lab exposure to blast overpressure. Cell death increased over time in cells closer to articular surfaces, and the investigators suggested that these changes might contribute to posttraumatic arthritis in blast-injured limbs. Using a rat model, Hurtgen et al., 2016, found that volumetric muscle loss injury impaired adjacent tibial healing after open fracture and was associated with specific immune system responses that might be targeted for prevention of delayed bone healing after severe traumatic injury.

We identified a few basic science studies conducted on animals to investigate surgical techniques that may aid in limb salvage. Siemionow et al., 2017, demonstrated the efficacy of the epineural sheath jacket to prevent neuroma in rat sciatic nerves. Neuromas are often painful in limb-salvage patients and hinder quality of life; it is possible that this technique could be used in this patient population to improve functionality following injury. Ward, Ji, and Corona, 2015, showed that autologous minced muscle grafts can be used to treat volumetric muscle loss, a common problem in orthopedic trauma. The researchers found that autologous minced grafts can be volume-expanded in a collagen hydrogel and that 50-percent minced graph tissue suspended in a collagen hydrogel was associated with a functional improvement similar to that of a 100-percent minced graft repair. However, more research is needed to identify optimal carrier materials for expansion. Garg et al., 2015, demonstrated, in a rat "open fracture" model, that volumetric loss of skeletal muscle results in persistent functional deficits that depend on muscle length and joint angle.

Clinical Research

In this section, we review the outcomes of limb-salvage procedures and subsequent recovery intervention strategies. There are four major studies of limb-salvage treatment outcomes: the Major Extremity Trauma Research Consortium (METRC), Lower Extremity Assessment Project (LEAP), Military Extremity Trauma Amputation/Limb Salvage (METALS) project, and U.S. Department of Veterans Affairs (VA) Vascular Injury Study (VAVIS). Although these projects are not specifically concerned with blast-related limb salvage and recovery, they are large prospective treatment studies that have shaped much of the scholarly discourse on the topic. In the following section, we summarize these landmark studies and what is known from these and other treatment research studies.

Seminal Studies on Amputation and Limb Salvage
LEAP (Lower Extremity Assessment Project)

The LEAP study, a prospective, multicenter observational study, focused on clarifying the decision to amputate or salvage a limb when there was severe lower-extremity trauma. The researchers attempted to define characteristics of individuals who sustained these types of injuries, the environment surrounding these injuries, and the physical aspects of these injuries. The study also defined the secondary medical and mental conditions that arose from these injuries and their treatments and looked at ultimate functional status and general health of the patients. The main finding from this study was that, while two-year outcomes were similar between limb-salvage patients and those who opted for amputation, limb-salvage patients were more likely to be rehospitalized in that two-year period (Bosse et al., 2002). The researchers evaluated all participants using the Sickness Impact Profile and found that predictors of a high (worse) score included rehospitalization for a major complication, low level of education, nonwhite race, poverty, lack of private health insurance, poor social-support network, low self-efficacy (the patient's confidence in being able to resume life activities), smoking, and involvement in disability-compensation litigation (Bosse et al., 2002).

METALS (Military Extremity Trauma Amputation/Limb Salvage)

The METALS study was a retrospective cohort study that included 324 service members deployed to Afghanistan or Iraq who had sustained a severe lower-limb injury requiring either limb salvage, surgery, or amputation. The study defined *limb salvage surgery* as involving revascularization, bone graft or bone transport, local or free flap coverage, repair of a major nerve injury, or a complete compartment injury or compartment syndrome. The study measured function, depression, posttraumatic stress disorder (PTSD), chronic pain, and engagement in sports and leisure activities. Using the Short Musculoskeletal Function Assessment, the researchers found that, in terms of function, patients had worse outcomes than population norms (except arm and hand scores). The researchers also found that 38.3 percent of patients screened positive for depressive symptoms, 17.9 percent screened positive for PTSD, and 34 percent were not working, were on active duty, or were in school (Doukas et al., 2013). Patients treated with amputation had better functional outcomes than those who had salvaged limbs. These patients also had a lower likelihood of PTSD and a higher likelihood of being engaged in "vigorous sports" (Doukas et al., 2013).

Currently, METRC is conducting ongoing analysis of both the LEAP and METALS studies and is seeking to compare and contrast the similarities and differences of both studies and to advance evidence-based patient-centered care (Rispoli and MacKenzie, 2012).

METRC (Major Extremity Trauma Research Consortium)

The METRC is a multisite clinical trials consortium that conducts studies relevant to the treatment and outcomes of orthopedic trauma sustained by military service members. The consortium includes more than 60 civilian trauma centers and four military treatment centers used to recruit patients; as of 2018, METRC was funded to conduct 32 prospective studies. The consortium was driven by five criteria when designing, selecting, and supporting studies: Studies had to (1) be multicenter, (2) be multidisciplinary, (3) be coordinated with the consortium to ensure quality, (4) address gaps in the research, and (5) have a sustainable approach (MacKenzie et al., 2017). Stinner et al., 2017, emphasized the importance of including civilian trauma centers; the researchers pointed out that the volume of participants needed to make more-conclusive discoveries was only possible by including civilian trauma centers in the study because combat casualty flow was episodic (Stinner et al., 2017). METRC has been successful at doing this (Major Extremity Trauma Research Consortium, 2016).

The work from the consortium is ongoing, and the researchers have developed a standardized set of measurement instruments to examine outcomes. These measurements cut across a defined set of key domains and include complications, depression, PTSD, pain, activity and participation, health-related quality of life, patient satisfaction, and health care utilization. The researchers have also developed a standardized collection of sociodemographic and clinical covariates, which will be collected across all studies (Castillo, MacKenzie, and Bosse, 2012). Results were not published during the study period for this review.

VAVIS (VA Vascular Injury Study)

The VAVIS is a longitudinal cohort study of veterans who have vascular extremity injuries. Although the study is not specifically about limb salvage, it will collect information critical to understanding long-term outcomes among limb-salvage patients. Critically, the researchers will be characterizing the preventive services received by individuals with vascular repair and the related outcomes of those services and describing patient-reported functional outcomes (Shireman et al., 2015). Although this study is promising, it has not yet produced results at the time of this review.

Surgical Approaches

Several reviews provide instruction relating to limb salvage–related techniques for surgeons and other clinicians. These reviews address, for example, lower-extremity reconstruction (Friedrich, Katolik, and Hanel, 2011; Soltanian, Garcia, and Hollenbeck, 2015); calcaneus fractures (Balazs et al., 2014); flap-based reconstruction (Friedrich, Katolik, and Hanel, 2011; Sabino, Slater, and Valerio, 2016; Soltanian, Garcia, and Hollenbeck, 2015); and blast-related foot injuries (Balazs et al., 2014; Keeling et al., 2010). Limb salvage–related surgical procedures typically are led by orthopedic surgeons; however, depending on the nature of the injury, vascular, neurosurgical, and particularly plastic surgeons play significant roles (Boriani et al., 2017).

When limb salvage is conducted, proper steps should be taken to ensure that, when appropriate, external fixators are used and wound debridements are repeated until a stable soft tissue envelope suitable for reconstruction is achieved (Blair et al., 2016). In this section, we discuss published research on related surgical approaches to provide an overview.

Flap construction is a major issue in limb salvage. In a meta-analysis of free flap surgery for combat injuries, the authors found that dorsi flaps were the most commonly used and that the success rate was 95.5 percent (Theodorakopoulou et al., 2016). With regard to blast-related limb salvage specifically, Sabino, Slater, and Valerio, 2016, discussed in their review that reconstruction—including free flap as the most-commonly used technique—conducted more than seven days after the injury allowed for patient stabilization and for the wound bed to be prepared. This is because blast injuries often have debris from the surrounding environment in the wound. The researchers also found that free tissue transfer had a high success rate in providing tissue outside the zone of injury while covering important structures for form and function. Finally, their review found that outcomes of fasiciocutaneous flaps were comparable to outcomes of muscle flaps, even after considering serious complications, such as proximal vascular injury, high platelet counts, and previous antifibrinolytic use (Sabino, Slater, and Valerio, 2016).

Another overview of approaches to foot injuries from blasts specifically made a note that a sufficient fat pad and range of motion were critical to the success of salvage surgeries if a service member wished to return to duty (Keeling et al., 2010). The researchers made the point when summarizing the cases they reviewed that a good result for the terminus of the salvaged foot was critical to the overall success of the salvage attempt (Keeling et al., 2010).

In an uncontrolled follow-up study, Dickson et al., 2015, followed 22 civilian adult patients (mean age 35, ranging from 17 to 64) with grade 3 open tibial fractures from traffic-, fall-, or crush-related accidental injuries for a year after external fixation using a circular frame. Of these patients, 36 percent went on to experience problems with walking and 14 percent had difficulties with independent self-care; 41 percent reported chronic pain, and 14 percent reported anxiety and depression. The researchers concluded, based on a review of previous studies, that circular frame fixation provided "good functional outcomes in the majority of cases" (Dickson et al., 2015, p. 751).

Surgical Level and Subsequent Outcome

Amputation may occur to different anatomical levels that typically are determined by the injury, and it is important to consider these differences when comparing the success of amputation procedures with that of limb-salvage procedures. Types of amputation may include foot, including toes or partial foot; at the ankle (ankle disarticulation); below the knee (transtibial); at the knee (knee disarticulation); above the knee (transfemoral); and at the hip (hip disarticulation). Amputation and salvage can be bilateral (both legs) or unilateral (one leg). Tintle et al., 2010, state that as much limb length as possible should be maintained without compromising healing or leaving painful residual limb or poor soft issue coverage. Studies suggests that osseous integration technology as related to the complex blast injury patient with a deficient residual limb has become an established clinical treatment option with substantial benefits for patients with lower-limb amputation (Frölke, Leijendekkers, and van de Meent, 2017; Hebert, Rehani, and Stiegelmar, 2017; Isaacson et al., 2010).

All of the studies we identified focused on lower-limb amputation versus salvage, and most studies examined multiple or unspecified levels or degrees of amputation and salvage. The most-common specified levels of amputation and reconstruction were transtibial (Penn-Barwell et al., 2015; Saddawi-Konefka, Kim, and Chung, 2008; Wilken et al., 2018) and foot (Bennett et al., 2018; Sheean, Krueger, and Hsu, 2014). Those who underwent transtibial amputation were significantly more likely to return to active duty than those who underwent all other amputation levels (Krueger and Wenke, 2014). Most studies focused on unilateral amputation or reconstruction, although one study clearly included patients with bilateral amputation or reconstruction (Bennett et al., 2018).

The number of studies we found was small, making it difficult to draw reliable conclusions; however, we could not identify a clear difference between outcomes of amputation and limb salvage, nor did we identify changes in this finding based on the extent of injury.

Surgical Timing and Subsequent Outcome

Limb salvage is an ongoing process, and amputation may occur at any point during the initial hospitalization or later. We found that the definition of *late amputation* varied across studies. Late amputation could refer to any time after the initial hospitalization, after a reconstruction procedure, or after another defined period—typically, three months. For example, studies used after 12 weeks (Huh et al., 2011) or after 90 days (Melcer et al., 2013) to define late amputation. Patients who receive late amputation tend to have worse mental and physical health outcomes, greater pain, and more complications compared with patients who receive early amputation, perhaps because patients receiving late amputation typically have failed earlier treatments (Melcer et al., 2017). Research has found that common reasons for late amputation in upper extremities include loss of wrist or finger motion, neurological pain, and heterotopic ossification (Krueger et al., 2014). One study found that early and delayed lower-limb amputation achieve similar results, suggesting that the watchful waiting approach to amputation might be reasonable (van der Merwe et al., 2016).

Complications After Surgery

Initial surgery for limb injury, whether amputation or reconstruction, can result in complications, such as tissue infection, osteomyelitis (bone infection), flap failure (unsuccessful tissue transfer), anemia, septicemia, thromboembolic disease, osteoporosis, or the need for rehospitalization. Additional complications can arise because of general complications following surgery, such as bleeding, reaction to anesthesia, and difficulty breathing.

Patients who undergo initial reconstruction may have additional complications, such as nonunion (bone healing complications), and might eventually need to undergo late amputation. In a systematic review of patients with IIIB and IIIC tibial fractures, complications after reconstruction included osteomyelitis (17.9 percent), nonunion (15.5 percent), secondary amputation (7.3 percent), and flap failure (5.8 percent) (Saddawi-Konefka, Kim, and Chung, 2008). The authors note that secondary amputation decreased with time across studies, likely because of improved salvage procedures, but that other rates of other complications have remained stable.

In contrast, patients who undergo amputation may have the additional complication of phantom limb syndrome, in which pain or other sensations are experienced in the amputated limb. In a retrospective review of patients injured in the wars in Iraq and Afghanistan, this complication was observed in 56 percent of amputees (Melcer et al., 2013).

In comparing relevant complications between initial amputation patients and reconstruction patients, results were mixed. Studies have found that patients who underwent initial amputation had lower rates of rehospitalization (Bosse et al., 2002), fewer subsequent surgeries (Bosse et al., 2002), and shorter hospital stays (Barla et al., 2017). By contrast, another study found that amputees had nearly double the risk of complications, including anemia, septicemia, and thromboembolic disease (Melcer et al., 2013). Amputees also had a higher risk of osteoporosis at one year post-injury, although there were no significant differences between the two groups in later years (Melcer et al., 2017).

Infections After Surgery

Our review of the wound infection literature relating to limb salvage was not exhaustive; note that blast injury–related wound infections were the focus of the sixth DoD SoSM (DoD Blast Injury Research Program Coordinating Office, 2016a; 2016b).

Studies have found conflicting or insignificant results linking limb-salvage procedures to infection and wound healing. Some research found lower overall infection rates following amputation than following limb reconstruction (Barla et al., 2017; Bosse et al., 2002), while other research found higher rates (Melcer et al., 2013). One study found no difference in osteomyelitis between groups and no difference in nonhealing wounds (Melcer et al., 2013). Another study found lower rates of osteomyelitis after amputation (Bosse et al., 2002).

One literature review found that, among combat injuries, the infection rates among open lower-limb fractures were similar to or higher than rates in the civilian population, although reports varied widely, from 23 to 85 percent (Rivera, Wenke, and Pugh, 2016). Of note, this review included studies of injuries that were not blast related. Another study found that most wounds had low-virulence, environmental gram-negative bacteria at initial testing that were not found again during therapy (Wallum et al., 2015). This study found a high incidence of contamination with environmental organisms that were not associated with infections during the course of the patient's care (Wallum et al., 2015). Ongoing work by Bosse and O'Toole might add to the understanding of infection management among blast-related limb-salvage patients (Bosse et al., 2017; O'Toole et al., 2017).

Pain After Surgery

Pain outcomes are a substantial consideration for many patients and can occur regardless of treatment course. Importantly, long-term pain after limb salvage ultimately can lead patients to the decision to amputate. In a study of British service members with combat-related hindfoot injuries, pain was cited as the most common reason (68 percent) for late amputation after initial reconstruction (Bennett et al., 2018).

Studies generally found lower levels of pain among patients who underwent amputation compared with those who underwent reconstruction, although these differences appeared to dissipate over time. In a retrospective, observational study of individuals with traumatic limb injuries, individuals with amputations reported lower levels of pain compared with patients with limb salvage (Ladlow et al., 2016). However, these differences might dissipate over time; the researchers found the prevalence of pain to be very low in both groups and differences to be no longer statistically significant following hospital discharge. Similarly, Penn-Barwell et al., 2015, found no significant long-term differences in prevalence of pain between those who underwent amputation and those who underwent limb salvage. In another long-term study of outcomes between patients with reconstruction and amputation, there were no significant differences in any pain diagnosis between the groups at four years, although patients who underwent amputation had significantly lower rates of osteoarthritis, specifically (Melcer et al., 2017).

Psychosocial Status After Surgery

Poor short- and long-term mental health outcomes are frequent following traumatic injury, and this is especially true for individuals who have sustained combat-related injuries. As previously noted by Young-McCaughan et al., 2017, service members with combat-related extremity trauma were assessed for pain, sleep disturbance, depression, and anxiety using validated measures at the time of hospital discharge. Eighty-eight percent had significant levels of pain, sleep disturbance, depression, or anxiety, and these symptomatic patients manifested mental health–related functioning roughly two standard deviations below population norms. Another large meta-analysis measured the prevalence of PTSD and depression in patients after major orthopedic trauma, finding that, of 7,109 participants, 32.6 percent experienced depression and 26.6 percent experienced PTSD (Muscatelli et al., 2017). Another study, Archer et al., 2016, reported that PTSD and depression were significantly associated with increased levels of pain at discharge from the hospital for patients with major orthopedic trauma to a limb. Additionally, in a case series analysis of individuals who had undergone late amputation following limb salvage, poor mental health and dissatisfaction with limb reconstruction were cited as reasons for undergoing late amputation in the majority of patients (Krueger et al., 2015).

Findings of mental health differences between patients with initial limb salvage and early amputation are mixed. In some studies comparing mental health outcomes between initial amputation and reconstructive surgery, there were no differences between groups. No differences in mental health were observed as measured by the Short-Form 12-item (SF-12) Mental Component Score (MCS) (Barla et al., 2017), the SF-36 MCS (Penn-Barwell et al., 2015), or the Sickness Impact Profile (SIP) (Bosse et al., 2002). Similarly, no differences in anxiety and depression (Ladlow et al., 2016) or the prevalence of PTSD (Melcer et al., 2017) were observed. However, one study of service members with combat-related hindfoot injuries found a higher prevalence of associated psychiatric-disabling conditions among patients who received reconstruction compared with those who received amputation (Sheean, Krueger, and Hsu, 2014). A meta-analysis of 11 studies comparing functional status in 769 patients with severe ("mangled") lower-limb injury who received amputation and 369 patients who received reconstructive surgery found a small, but significant, difference favoring reconstructive surgery patients in terms of psychological functioning, but found no significant difference in physical functioning (Akula et al., 2011).

The management of recovery expectations might be especially difficult after patients have undergone reconstructive limb-salvage surgery. Readiness to Engage in Self-Management After Acute Traumatic Injury (RESMATI) is an instrument conceptually based on a stages-of-change model. The RESMATI is potentially a good instrument to evaluate injured patients' readiness to engage in self-motivated recovery efforts (e.g., increased activation and accessing relationships and learning resources) (Wegener et al., 2014). The Trauma Collaborative Care program, an intervention based on the principles of collaborative care, could also be a good model to help patients manage their own psychological care (Wegener et al., 2017). Most of these findings are not related specifically to limb salvage per se, and mental health issues can occur regardless of whether the limb is amputated or salvaged. However, as it relates to limb salvage, the management of recovery expectations might be especially difficult after patients have undergone reconstructive surgery. In the short term, pastoral care, teaching coping skills and mindfulness, peer education, and access to educational resources have been shown to be effective at mitigating some of the mental health issues following orthopedic trauma. In the long term, peer networks, such as the Trauma Survivors Network, have been shown to be effective (Vincent et al., 2015).

Functional Status After Surgery

Studies have shown that patients who underwent amputation had shorter time until full weight bearing (Saddawi-Konefka, Kim, and Chung, 2008), could walk greater distances, were more likely to be able to run (Ladlow et al., 2016), and had fewer gait deficiencies with more time spent on the affected limb (Mangan et al., 2016) compared with those who underwent reconstructive surgery. However, another study that examined longer-term mobility (an average of two years following surgery)—as measured by sit-to-stand, four-square step, and timed stair-ascent tests—found no difference between patients who underwent amputation and those who underwent limb salvage (Wilken et al., 2018).

One study found higher physical functioning scores, as measured by the Physical Component Score (PCS), among those who underwent amputation (Bennett et al., 2018), but other studies found no difference in physical function scores as measured by the SF-36 PCS (Bennett et al., 2018) and SIP (Bosse et al., 2002) between those who underwent amputation and those who underwent reconstruction.

Return-to-work results likewise were mixed, with one study finding faster return-to-work among amputees (Saddawi-Konefka, Kim, and Chung, 2008) and another study, focused only on service members, finding that those who underwent reconstruction had lower levels of disability and were more likely to return to duty (Sheean, Krueger, and Hsu, 2014). One study also found shorter rehabilitation times for limb-salvage patients, compared with amputees (Ladlow et al., 2016).

In sum, these comparisons of physical functioning outcomes between patients who have undergone amputation and those who have undergone reconstructive surgery have yielded mixed results. The majority of studies that we identified found better outcomes in terms of mobility among patients who underwent amputation shortly after surgery, but little difference was observed for other functional outcomes.

Costs of Care After Surgery

Although we did not identify high-quality evidence that consistently favored either amputation or limb salvage after severe limb injury, the largest differences might be related to costs. Indeed, one study projected lifetime health care costs that were nearly three times higher for amputation than for reconstructive surgery (MacKenzie et al., 2007).

Costs initially appear similar for both procedures; the MacKenzie et al., 2007, study found no difference in initial hospitalization costs between groups. However, amputation involved more-costly prostheses and higher lifetime medical costs (MacKenzie et al., 2007). Another study found that, even disregarding prostheses costs, lifetime medical costs were higher for those with amputation (Chung et al., 2009).

Surgical Decisions and Decision Aids for Treatment Selection

After severe high-energy or blast-related limb injury, both clinicians and patients often are faced with difficult decisions about when to amputate the injured extremity versus when to salvage and reconstruct it. There is general recognition that clinicians should have ongoing discussions about treatment options and risks with the patient and, as appropriate, family members or other representatives of the patient (Aravind, Shauver, and Chung, 2010).

The appropriate course of action is not always clear, and many have attempted to summarize the factors involved in these decisions

(Blair et al., 2016; Langer, 2014). Clinical factors often favoring amputation include (1) when the extremity is avulsed (i.e., skin and soft tissue are partially or completely torn away), (2) bony damage that cannot be surgically reconstructed, (3) severe combined injuries, and (4) warm ischemia time of more than six hours, resulting in extensive soft tissue necrosis (Brown et al., 2011). However, predicting outcome after severe blast-related extremity injury remains an inexact science. Hanson-Viana et al., 2018, illustrates the challenges, describing a young, healthy adult male who suffered a severe fireworks injury resulting in a poor-prognosis popliteal vascular injury after some 12 hours of "hot" ischemia. An end-to-end anastomosis (reattachment) of the popliteal vein and arterial repair were performed, and, at six months, the patient's scars had healed and he was ambulating with a walking aid and "minimal limitations of knee movement" (Hanson-Viana et al., 2018). Research in civilian trauma centers found that amputation was significantly more common in lower extremities when the patient suffered a blunt anterior tibia vessel injury as opposed to a posterior tibial or peroneal injury (Scalea et al., 2014).

Outcomes of importance when deciding whether to amputate or salvage a limb after a blast or severe high-energy trauma exposure include survival; risk of surgical complications, including infection; functional and cosmetic outcomes; short- and long-term pain and psychosocial outcomes; and health care costs. A guiding principle in selecting limb salvage should be that the expected functional outcome for the patient will be at least as good as a best-level amputation. Outcomes change over time, and both short- and long-term perspectives should be considered. To our knowledge, no randomized controlled trials have been reported to compare the results of amputation with those of limb salvage or reconstruction. Prospective and retrospective observational studies have been conducted (Saddawi-Konefka, Kim, and Chung, 2008). Assessing the link between intervention and an outcome in observational studies involves substantial uncertainty, although a few studies have attempted to control for potentially confounding factors, such as injury, patient, and environmental characteristics. An extensive review on the decision to amputate versus salvage the limb has been completed by Rush, Arrington, and Hsu, 2012.

Although Dua et al., 2014, studied 68 patients with popliteal artery trauma and found that patients with a Mangled Extremity Severity Score (MESS) greater than 7 had an increased likelihood of amputation, Balci et al., 2015, found that the MESS score had limited capacity as an amputation decision aid and instead recommended careful conversation with patients before deciding on amputation versus limb salvage on clinical grounds. Brown et al., 2011, and Momoh and Chung, 2013, also concluded that the MESS lacked predictive utility.

Measures that predict outcomes that could aid clinical decisions to amputate or salvage a severely injured limb are lacking (Cross and Swiontkowski, 2011). For patients who have already undergone limb-salvage surgery, the Short Musculoskeletal Function Assessment (SMFA), a 46-item self-report instrument, quantitatively assesses functional status following orthopedic trauma. Scott et al., 2014, employed the SMFA for use in patients after vascular injury to an extremity. In a sample of 84 civilians with previous lower-limb injuries, Teicher et al., 2014, found the SMFA score was predictive of whether patients were likely to need future surgical procedures, develop more medical complications, or require a longer hospital stay; most of the predictive effect was among infected patients. Surgeons recommend clinical considerations and regular, realistic discussions with patients as opposed to reliance on a scoring system to determine the best course of treatment (Tunali et al., 2017). Momoh and Chung, 2013, conducted a detailed review of preoperative scoring systems to identify patients who would benefit from early amputation and concluded that there was insufficient evidence to suggest that any of the several instruments previously studied were up to the task.

Numerous assessments have been used in longitudinal studies of limb salvage to track mobility and physical function. Williams, Hill, and Kahn, 2014, developed the High-Level Mobility Assessment Tool (HiMAT) to assess patients following severe lower-limb trauma ("multitrauma"), comparing findings to those obtained using the Functional Independence Measure (FIM) and the Lower Extremity Functional Scale (LEFS). The investigators reported that the HiMAT was more responsive and less susceptible to ceiling effects than the FIM and LEFS and was not well correlated with FIM and LEFS, suggesting that it might be measuring somewhat different aspects of functioning and mobility (Williams, Hill, and Kahn, 2014). A study of a subsequent version of the HiMAT suggested that the measure was a unidimensional assessment of high mobility with good construct validity and minimal floor and ceiling effects (Hill et al., 2014). LEFS has been successfully used to demonstrate functionality following free tissue transfer surgery (i.e., dissection and detachment of vascularized tissue from one region of the body and transfer and reattachment to another body region) (Falola et al., 2018). Of note, the reliability and validity of these assessments in patients with severe blast-related extremity injuries is unknown. Although there are more than 100 mobility measurement tools (Bushnell et al., 2015), to our knowledge, there has not been an evidence-based recommendation of which tool to use to measure long-term functioning and mobility after limb trauma surgery or interventions.

In a retrospective case-control study, Petfield et al., 2017, investigated the impact on clinical management of virtual stress testing (VST) for 65 military patients with tibial fractures treated using external fixation. VST is a noninvasive test that uses computed tomography (CT) to estimate the strength of healing bone tissue. Using post-hoc thresholds, the researchers were able to accurately identify all of the nine patients who failed the treatment and about three-fourths of those with an uneventful recovery after removal of the external fixator (Petfield et al., 2017). In a small, uncontrolled study of patients seen after high-energy tibial plafond fractures, LeBus and Collinge performed computed tomographic angiography (CTA), finding that the procedure identified significant distal arterial abnormalities in slightly more than half of patients. They concluded that CTA was safe and potentially useful in this preoperative context (LeBus and Collinge, 2008).

Prospective, observational evidence suggests that, in the short term, amputation might offer patients better pain and functional status outcomes than reconstructive surgery to salvage the limb (Bosse et al., 2002). However, these benefits might dissipate over time. In the LEAP study, one of the largest studies of patients with severe leg injuries, patients underwent either amputation or reconstructive surgery and were followed for seven years. Although patients who underwent amputations had better outcomes initially, there was no significant difference between the two groups in functional health outcomes after two years, even after adjusting for potential confounders, including patient demographics and injury characteristics (Bosse et al., 2002); results were similar at seven-year follow-up (MacKenzie et al., 2005).

Rehabilitative Approaches

In perhaps the most-widely cited study of combat-related extremity trauma treatment, patients treated with amputation had better functional outcomes than those who had salvaged limbs (Doukas et al., 2013). Early mobilization and strength training are fundamental to rehabilitation (Hoyt et al., 2015). Rehabilitation of the patient with limb salvage was not as focused as it was for the patient with amputation until the development of the dynamic ankle-foot orthosis (AFO) and the Return to Run (RTR) clinical pathway. A signature contribution to the limb-salvage patient from Operation Iraqi Freedom and Operation Enduring Freedom was likely the transition of prosthetic fabrication techniques and advanced carbon-fiber materials from the amputation sector to orthotic development for the limb-salvage patient with residual limb dysfunction. The rehabilitation pathway involves early intervention in the limb-salvage patient's recovery, with a focus on strength, horizontal plyometrics, and run retraining. Once the surgeon authorizes full weight bearing, the patient is fitted with a dynamic AFO and progresses to more-high-energy exercises, vertical plyometrics, strength and agility conditioning, and run retraining. It takes, on average, 12 weeks to complete the program (Owens et al., 2011). Sheean et al., 2016, found positive results using the RTR program among active-duty service members with severe lower-limb trauma. Participants in their study had improved physical performance and patient-reported outcomes. A systematic literature review concluded that the RTR program coupled with a dynamic AFO "can enable return to duty, return to recreation and physical activity and decrease pain in some high functioning patients" (Highsmith et al., 2016). Another study found that just more than 19 percent of service members wishing to return to their previous duty were able to do so after the RTR program (Patzkowski, Owens, et al., 2012). Potter et al., 2018, showed a significant improvement in the SMFA score of limb-salvage patients fitted with and trained to use the dynamic AFO (Frölke, Leijendekkers, and van de Meent, 2017; Potter et al., 2018).

Crowell et al., 2016, showed clinically meaningful changes in self-reported function and improvements to physical performance when using orthopedic manual physical therapy in addition to the RTR clinical pathway. However, the study only included three participants and so was unable to demonstrate any statistically significant results. More research is needed in this area.

Prosthetics and Orthotics

A number of prosthetics, which replace body parts (such as amputated limbs), and orthoses, which support or align body parts (particularly in the case of reconstructive limbs), have been developed or improved. Only one study, which compared the limb-salvage population to the amputee population, specified type of orthosis used. In a study of military trauma patients with unilateral lower-limb injuries, patients with amputation had better walking outcomes, including faster gait and more time spent on the affected limb, compared with patients in the reconstruction group, who completed a special training program and used a dynamic AFO (Mangan et al., 2016).

Exoskeletal Devices

Physical therapy may incorporate the use of orthotic devices to assist with rehabilitation and improve long-term function. Bedigrew et al., 2014, found that integrating the use of a dynamic AFO improved physical performance, pain, and patient-reported outcomes; however, there was no comparison group in this study. The dynamic AFO also was tested as a device to help navigate stairs. Authors found that the device helps users navigate stairs unassisted (Whitehead, Esposito, and Wilken, 2016). Patzkowski, Blanck, et al., 2012, found that the patients receiving the dynamic AFO manifested better performance on validated tests of agility, power, and speed, compared with patients with no brace.

CHAPTER FOUR

Discussion and Recommendations

The review of recent literature on limb salvage and recovery after severe blast injury was intended to facilitate the eighth SoSM, a process undertaken to determine topic-specific DoD research priorities. To focus our review conclusions and to facilitate the practical use of these conclusions in formulating research directions and priorities, we break the conclusions down to address each of the four main literature review objectives. For each objective, we discuss our findings and offer recommendations.

Describe the Epidemiology and Outcomes of Limb Salvage After Severe Blast-Related Limb Injury

Findings

We found that severe limb injuries were common among combat-injured service members—even more common than in the blast-injured subpopulation—and that most of these injuries were from explosive munitions. Subsequent symptoms include persistent pain, sleep disturbance, depression and anxiety, and general loss of functioning. These symptoms remain persistent and disabling, even after substantial rehabilitative care, and medical complications are common. Although a significant minority of service members have returned to duty after severe blast-related limb injuries, the vast majority with severe combat-related limb injury are significantly and permanently disabled (Sheean, Krueger, and Hsu, 2014). The near absence of completed prospective, longitudinal studies with follow-up longer than one year is an important gap.

Recommendations

To characterize the occurrence of severe blast-related limb injuries in a combat theater, the rapid, early establishment of theater-wide medical surveillance systems (e.g., Military Orthopaedic Trauma Registry) and studies with multiyear follow-up are needed. Identifying injuries in this manner will lead to opportunities to better validate outcome measures, estimate rates of complications, improve prognostication methods, identify optimal candidates for limb-salvage efforts, and initiate prospective, longitudinal cohort studies with long follow-up.

Review the Evidence About the Decision to Salvage Versus Amputate a Limb After a Severe Blast-Related Limb Injury

Findings

To date, prognostic assessment tools have largely failed as decision aids for clinicians and patients. A consensus of expert clinicians has suggested that there is no one-size-fits-all intervention approach to severe blast-related limb injuries and that ongoing, intensive efforts to share and study decisionmaking with patients, caregivers (as appropriate), and a multidisciplinary clinical team are needed. Treatment planning should be patient-centered and account for the patient's perspective and addressing patient-reported objectives and needs (Aravind, Shauver, and Chung, 2010). Furthermore, there is limited evidence on the outcomes of amputation patients versus limb-salvage patients who encountered blasts specifically. This is problematic because blast-related limb-salvage patients are more likely to have complications, such as infection, than non-blast-related severe limb-injury patients. Better evidence to guide decisionmaking is needed and efforts to accumulate evidence during peacetime might be necessary.

Recommendations

During peace, longitudinal studies and controlled clinical trials that address decisionmaking and clarify the relative merits of limb salvage versus amputation should recruit patients from the vast U.S. network of civilian trauma centers. Although classical blast-related injury in these settings is less than common, patients with other high-energy mechanisms of severe traumatic limb injury (e.g., motor vehicle accidents) can be recruited from multiple centers in numbers that could make innovative and potentially convincing controlled trial research designs possible.

Future research should explore feasible clinical models of shared decisionmaking, patient-centered treatment planning, and patient-reported outcomes pertaining to limb salvage–related decisions following severe limb trauma. Military hospitals should partner with civilian trauma centers and extremity trauma clinical research platforms to strengthen research ties and investigate the impact of military clinician training in these settings on the development and maintenance of limb salvage–related skills among military clinicians.

Examine Evidence and Innovations About Restoration and Reconstruction After Limb Salvage for Severe Blast-Related Limb Injury

Findings

Current evidence comparing various surgical approaches to limb salvage for blast-related limb injury is preliminary at best.

Recommendations

As new salvage techniques are introduced, we recommend that a series of a large, multicenter trials enrolling civilians is instituted. Depending on the military tempo of combat operations occurring in parallel with these studies, it might be possible to include patients with high-energy sources of severe limb injuries from both military and civilian populations. This multicenter approach will maximize the likelihood of enrolling enough patients to obtain adequate statistical power to identify clinically important differences in outcomes when comparing treatment strategies.

Review Evidence and Innovations About Rehabilitation, Reintegration, and Recovery After Limb Salvage for Severe Blast-Related Limb Injury

Findings

The most underdeveloped area of empirical research we reviewed pertained to rehabilitative approaches for the care of blast-injured patients with severe limb injuries. Promising programs have been identified (e.g., RTR program, dynamic AFO device), but more-robust efforts to codify and empirically evaluate these complex interventions and emerging technologies are needed. Studies evaluating an early and universal application of a dynamic AFO to the at-risk limb-salvage patient are needed to better determine the efficacy and clinical impact of the modern orthotic.

Recommendations

We recommend researching complex multidisciplinary rehabilitation and reintegration strategies to support service members and their caregivers in achieving recovery and possibly a return to military service. We recommend—similar to the research strategies for limb-salvage and reconstruction interventions in our third recommendation— codification of complex rehabilitative interventions for limb-salvage patients and exploration of the feasibility, important outcomes, assessments of intervention fidelity, and specific randomized designs that are most appropriate for studying the effectiveness of complex rehabilitative strategies. As for limb-salvage interventions (see the third recommendation), we recommend that a series of a large multicenter trials enrolling civilians be instituted. Again, it might be possible to include patients with high-energy sources of severe limb injuries from both military and civilian populations, but in the absence of military or VA opportunities to recruit participants, civilian rehabilitative care candidates with previous high-energy limb trauma injuries may provide reasonably generalizable results.

Rehabilitative psychosocial interventions that reduce service members' suffering from chronic pain, persistent sleep disorders, PTSD, anxiety, and related consequences of these injuries—consequences that can drive reductions in post-injury functioning—are essential, in addition to development and use of validated measures on limb strength, performance, and function.

Planning Committee Members

This meeting was made possible thanks to the guidance, planning, and insights of the members of the eighth SoSM planning committee.

Stuart Campbell
Extremity Trauma and Amputation Center of Excellence

Jill Cancio
Extremity Trauma and Amputation Center of Excellence,
Center for the Intrepid

Rory Cooper
University of Pittsburgh

Andrea Crunkhorn
Extremity Trauma and Amputation Center of Excellence

Christopher Dearth
Extremity Trauma and Amputation Center of Excellence

CAPT Eric Elster
Uniformed Services University of the Health Sciences

Alberto Esquenazi
Einstein Medical Center

Mike Galarneau
Naval Health Research Center

COL Brandon Goff
Center for the Intrepid

MAJ David Kingery
U.S. Army Institute of Surgical Research

Joe Miller
Extremity Trauma and Amputation Center of Excellence

LTC Keith Myers
Walter Reed National Military Medical Center

LTC Leon Nesti
Uniformed Services University/U.S. Army Medical Research and
Materiel Command

Benjamin Potter
Walter Reed National Military Medical Center

Lloyd Rose
U.S. Army Medical Research and Materiel Command, Clinical and
Rehabilitative Medicine Research Program

Daniel Stinner
Vanderbilt University Medical Center, Department of Orthopaedic
Surgery

Erik Wolf
U.S. Army Medical Research and Materiel Command

Anne Ritter
U.S. Army Medical Research and Materiel Command, Combat Casualty Care Research Program

References

Akula, Maheswara, Sreenadh Gella, C. J. Shaw, Phil McShane, and A. M. Mohsen, "A Meta-Analysis of Amputation Versus Limb Salvage in Mangled Lower Limb Injuries—The Patient Perspective," *Injury*, Vol. 42, No. 11, November 2011, pp. 1194–1197.

Aoki, Stephen Kenji, "Editorial Commentary: Hip Arthroscopy for Femoroacetabular Impingement: Outcomes May Be Depressing," *Arthroscopy: The Journal of Arthroscopic and Related Surgery*, Vol. 34, No. 8, August 2018, pp. 2375–2376.

Aravind, Maya, Melissa J. Shauver, and Kevin C. Chung, "A Qualitative Analysis of the Decision-Making Process for Patients with Severe Lower Leg Trauma," *Plastic and Reconstructive Surgery*, Vol. 126, No. 6, December 2010, pp. 2019–2029.

Archer, Kristin R., Sara E. Heins, Christine M. Abraham, William T. Obremskey, Stephen T. Wegener, and Renan C. Castillo, "Clinical Significance of Pain at Hospital Discharge Following Traumatic Orthopedic Injury: General Health, Depression, and PTSD Outcomes at 1 Year," *Clinical Journal of Pain*, Vol. 32, No. 3, March 2016, pp. 196–202.

Balazs, George C., Elizabeth M. Polfer, Alaina M. Brelin, and Wade T. Gordon, "High Seas to High Explosives: The Evolution of Calcaneus Fracture Management in the Military," *Military Medicine*, Vol. 179, No. 11, November 2014, pp. 1228–1235.

Balci, H. I., Y. Saglam, O. Tunali, T. Akgul, M. Aksoy, and F. Dikici, "Grade 3C Open Femur Fractures with Vascular Repair in Adults," *Acta Orthopaedica Belgica*, Vol. 81, No. 2, June 2015, pp. 274–282. As of April 6, 2020: https://www.ncbi.nlm.nih.gov/pubmed/26280967

Barla, M., B. Gavanier, M. Mangin, J. Parot, C. Bauer, and D. Mainard, "Is Amputation a Viable Treatment Option in Lower Extremity Trauma? *Orthopaedics & Traumatology, Surgery & Research*, Vol. 103, No. 6, October 2017, pp. 971–975.

Bedigrew, Katherine M., Jeanne C. Patzkowski, Jason M. Wilken, Johnny G. Owens, Ryan V. Blanck, Daniel J. Stinner, Kevin L. Kirk, Joseph R. Hsu, and Skeletal Trauma Research Consortium (STReC), "Can an Integrated Orthotic and Rehabilitation Program Decrease Pain and Improve Function After Lower Extremity Trauma?" *Clinical Orthopaedics and Related Research*, Vol. 472, No. 10, 2014, pp. 3017–3025.

Bennett, P. M., T. Stevenson, I. D. Sargeant, A. Mountain, and J. G. Penn-Barwell, "Outcomes Following Limb Salvage After Combat Hindfoot Injury Are Inferior to Delayed Amputation at Five Years," *Bone & Joint Research*, Vol. 7, No. 2, February 2018, pp. 131–138.

Blair, James A., Emmanuel D. Eisenstein, Sarah N. Pierrie, Wade Gordon, Johnny G. Owens, and Joseph R. Hsu, "Lower Extremity Limb Salvage: Lessons Learned from 14 Years at War," *Journal of Orthopaedic Trauma*, Vol. 30, Supplement 3, October 2016, pp. S11–S15.

Boriani, Filippo, Ata Ul Haq, Tommaso Baldini, Roberto Urso, Donatella Granchi, Nicola Baldini, Domenico Tigani, Moazzam Tarar, and Umraz Khan, "Orthoplastic Surgical Collaboration Is Required to Optimise the Treatment of Severe Limb Injuries: A Multi-Centre, Prospective Cohort Study," *Journal of Plastic, Reconstructive & Aesthetic Surgery*, Vol. 70, No. 6, June 2017, pp. 715–722.

Bosse, Michael J., Ellen J. MacKenzie, James F. Kellam, Andrew R. Burgess, Lawrence X. Webb, Marc F. Swiontkowski, Roy W. Sanders, Alan L. Jones, Mark P. McAndrew, Brendan M. Patterson, Melissa L. McCarthy, Thomas G. Travison, and Renan C. Castillo, "An Analysis of Outcomes of Reconstruction or Amputation After Leg-Threatening Injuries," *New England Journal of Medicine*, Vol. 347, No. 24, December 12, 2002, pp. 1924–1931.

Bosse, Michael J., Clinton K. Murray, Anthony R. Carlini, Reza Firoozabadi, Theodore Manson, Daniel O. Scharfstein, Joseph C. Wenke, Mary Zadnik, Renan C. Castillo, and METRC, "Assessment of Severe Extremity Wound Bioburden at the Time of Definitive Wound Closure or Coverage: Correlation with Subsequent Postclosure Deep Wound Infection (Bioburden Study)," *Journal of Orthopaedic Trauma*, Vol. 31, Supplement 1, April 2017, pp. S3–S9.

Brown, K. V., P. Henman, S. Stapley, and J. C. Clasper, J. C., "Limb Salvage of Severely Injured Extremities After Military Wounds," *Journal of the Royal Army Medical Corps*, Vol. 157, Supplement 3, September 2011, pp. S315–S323.

Bushnell, Cheryl, Janet Prvu Bettger, Kevin M. Cockroft, Steven C. Cramer, Maria Orlando Edelen, Daniel Hanley, Irene Katzan, Soeren Mattke, Dawn M. Nilsen, Tepring Piquado, Elizabeth R. Skidmore, Kay Wing, and Gayane Yenokyan, "Chronic Stroke Outcome Measures for Motor Function Intervention Trials: Expert Panel Recommendations," *Circulation: Cardiovascular Quality and Outcomes*, Vol. 8, No. 6, Supplement 3, October 2015, pp. S163–S169.

Castillo, Renan C., Ellen J. MacKenzie, and Michael J. Bosse on behalf of the METRC investigators, "Measurement of Functional Outcomes in the Major Extremity Trauma Research Consortium (METRC)," *Journal of the American Academy of Orthopaedic Surgeons*, Vol. 20, 2012, pp. S59–S63.

Chandler, Henry, Kirsty MacLeod, and Jowan G. Penn-Barwell, Severe Extremity Combat Trauma (SeLECT) Study Group, "Extremity Injuries Sustained by the UK Military in the Iraq and Afghanistan Conflicts: 2003–2014," *Injury*, Vol. 48, No. 7, July 2017, pp. 1439–1443.

Chung, Kevin C., Daniel Saddawi-Konefka, Steven C. Haase, and Gautam Kaul, "A Cost-Utility Analysis of Amputation Versus Salvage for Gustilo IIIB and IIIC Open Tibial Fractures," *Plastic and Reconstructive Surgery*, Vol. 124, No. 6, December 2009, pp. 1965–1973.

Cross, William W., III, and Marc F. Swiontkowski, "Outcome and Management of Primary Amputations, Subtotal Amputation Injuries, and Severe Open Fractures with Nerve Injuries," in Hans-Christoph Pape, Roy Sanders, and Joseph Borrelli, Jr., eds., *The Poly-Traumatized Patient with Fractures: A Multi-Disciplinary Approach*, 2nd ed., Heidelberg, Germany: Springer-Verlag Berlin Heidelberg, 2011, pp. 265–280.

Crowell, Michael S., Gail D. Deyle, Johnny Owens, and Norman W. Gill, "Manual Physical Therapy Combined with High-Intensity Functional Rehabilitation for Severe Lower Extremity Musculoskeletal Injuries: A Case Series," *Journal of Manual & Manipulative Therapy*, Vol. 24, No. 1, May 6, 2016 pp. 34–44.

Department of Defense Directive 6025.21E, *Medical Research for Prevention, Mitigation, and Treatment of Blast Injuries*, Washington, D.C.: Under Secretary of Defense for Research and Engineering, October 15, 2018. As of April 6, 2020: https://www.esd.whs.mil/Portals/54/Documents/DD/issuances/dodd/602521p. pdf?ver=2018-10-24-112151-983

Dickson, D. R., E. Moulder, Y. Hadland, P. V. Giannoudis, and H. K. Sharma, "Grade 3 Open Tibial Shaft Fractures Treated with a Circular Frame, Functional Outcome and Systematic Review of Literature," *Injury*, Vol. 46, No. 4, April 2015, pp. 751–758.

DoD—*See* U.S. Department of Defense.

DoD Blast Injury Research Program Coordinating Office—*See* U.S. Department of Defense Blast Injury Research Program Coordinating Office.

Doukas, William C., Roman A. Hayda, H. Michael Frisch, Romney C. Andersen, Michael T. Mazurek, James R. Ficke, John J. Keeling, Paul F. Pasquina, Harold J. Wain, Anthony R. Carlini, and Ellen J. MacKenzie, "The Military Extremity Trauma Amputation/Limb Salvage (METALS) Study: Outcomes of Amputation Versus Limb Salvage Following Major Lower-Extremity Trauma," *Journal of Bone & Joint Surgery*, Vol. 95, No. 2, January 2013, pp. 138–145.

Dua, Anahita, Sapan S. Desai, Jaecel O. Shah, Robert E. Lasky, Kristofer M. Charlton-Ouw, Ali Azizzadeh, Anthony L. Estrera, Hazim J. Safi, and Sheila M. Coogan, "Outcome Predictors of Limb Salvage in Traumatic Popliteal Artery Injury," *Annals of Vascular Surgery*, Vol. 28, No. 1, January 1, 2014, pp. 108–114.

Falola, Reuben A., Chrisovalantis Lakhiani, Jocelyn Green, Siya Patil, Brandon Jackson, Rachel Bratescu, Ersilia Anghel, John S. Steinberg, Paul J. Kim, Christopher E. Attinger, and Karen K. Evans, "Assessment of Function After Free Tissue Transfer to the Lower Extremity for Chronic Wounds Using the Lower Extremity Functional Scale," *Journal of Reconstructive Microsurgery*, Vol. 34, No. 5, June 2018, pp. 327–333.

Friedrich, J. B., L. I. Katolik, and D. P. Hanel, "Reconstruction of Soft-Tissue Injury Associated with Lower Extremity Fracture," *Journal of the American Academy of Orthopaedic Surgeons*, Vol. 19, No. 2, February 2011, pp. 81–90.

Frölke, J. P. M., R. A. Leijendekkers, H. van de Meent, "Osseointegrated Prosthesis for Patients with an Amputation," *Der Unfallchirurg*, Vol. 120, No. 4, 2017, pp. 293–299.

Garg, Koyal, Catherine L. Ward, Brady J. Hurtgen, Jason M. Wilken, Daniel J. Stinner, Joseph C. Wenke, Johnny G. Owens, and Benjamin T. Corona, "Volumetric Muscle Loss: Persistent Functional Deficits Beyond Frank Loss of Tissue," *Journal of Orthopaedic Research*, Vol. 33, No. 1, January 2015, pp. 40–46.

Hanson-Viana, Erik, Mónica González-Rodríguez, Diego García-Vivanco, and Mariel González-Calatayud, "Controversial Case: Revascularization of a Popliteal Vascular Injury of Poor Prognosis," *International Journal of Surgery Case Reports*, Vol. 49, 2018, pp. 185–190.

Hebert, Jacqueline S., Mayank Rehani, and Robert Stiegelmar, "Osseointegration for Lower-Limb Amputation: A Systematic Review of Clinical Outcomes," *JBJS Reviews*, Vol. 5, No. 10, October 2017, p. e10.

Highsmith, M. Jason, Leif M. Nelson, Neil T. Carbone, Tyler D. Klenow, Jason T. Kahle, Owen T. Hill, Jason T. Maikos, Mike S. Kartel, and Billie J. Randolph, "Outcomes Associated with the Intrepid Dynamic Exoskeletal Orthosis (IDEO): A Systematic Review of the Literature," *Military Medicine*, Vol. 181, November–December 2016, pp. 69–76.

Hill, Bridget, Michelle Kahn, Julie Pallant, and Gavin Williams, "Assessment of the Internal Construct Validity of the Revised High-Level Mobility Assessment Tool for Traumatic Orthopaedic Injuries," *Clinical Rehabilitation*, Vol. 28, No. 5, 2014, pp. 491–498.

Hoyt, Benjamin W., Gabriel J. Pavey, Paul F. Pasquina, and Benjamin K. Potter, "Rehabilitation of Lower Extremity Trauma: A Review of Principles and Military Perspective on Future Directions," *Current Trauma Reports*, Vol. 1, January 2015, pp. 50–60.

Huh, Jeannie, Daniel Stinner, Travis C. Burns, Joseph R. Hsu, and Late Amputation Study Team, "Infectious Complications and Soft Tissue Injury Contribute to Late Amputation After Severe Lower Extremity Trauma," *Journal of Trauma: Injury, Infection, and Critical Care*, Vol. 71, Supplement 1, July 2011, pp. S47–S51.

Hurtgen, B. J., C. L. Ward, K. Garg, B. E. Pollot, S. M. Goldman, T. O. McKinley, J. C. Wenke, and B. T. Corona, "Severe Muscle Trauma Triggers Heightened and Prolonged Local Musculoskeletal Inflammation and Impairs Adjacent Tibia Fracture Healing," *Journal of Musculoskeletal and Neuronal Interactions*, Vol. 16, No. 2, June 2016, pp. 122–134.

Isaacson, Brad M., Jeroen G. Stinstra, Rob S. MacLeod, Paul F. Pasquina, and Roy D. Bloebaum, "Developing a Quantitative Measurement System for Assessing Heterotopic Ossification and Monitoring the Bioelectric Metrics from Electrically Induced Osseointegration in the Residual Limb of Service Members," *Annals of Biomedical Engineering*, Vol. 38, No. 9, September 2010, pp. 2968–2978.

Keeling, John J., Joseph R. Hsu, Scott B. Shawen, and Romney C. Andersen, "Strategies for Managing Massive Defects of the Foot in High-Energy Combat Injuries of the Lower Extremity," *Foot and Ankle Clinics*, Vol. 15, No. 1, March 2010, pp. 139–149.

Krueger, Chad A., Jessica C. Rivera, David J. Tennent, Andrew J. Sheean, Daniel J. Stinner, and Joseph C. Wenke, "Late Amputation May Not Reduce Complications or Improve Mental Health in Combat-Related, Lower Extremity Limb Salvage Patients," *Injury*, Vol. 46, No. 8, August 2015, pp. 1527–1532.

Krueger, Chad A., and Joseph C. Wenke, "Initial Injury Severity and Social Factors Determine Ability to Deploy After Combat-Related Amputation," *Injury*, Vol. 45, No. 8, August 2014, pp. 1231–1235.

Krueger, Chad A., Joseph C. Wenke, Mickey S. Cho, and Joseph R. Hsu, "Common Factors and Outcome in Late Upper Extremity Amputations After Military Injury," *Journal of Orthopaedic Trauma*, Vol. 28, No. 4, April 2014, pp. 227–231.

Ladlow, Peter, Rhodri Phillip, Russell Coppack, John Etherington, James Bilzon, M. Polly McGuigan, and Alexander N. Bennett, "Influence of Immediate and Delayed Lower-Limb Amputation Compared with Lower-Limb Salvage on Functional and Mental Health Outcomes Post-Rehabilitation in the U.K. Military," *Journal of Bone & Joint Surgery*, Vol. 98, No. 23, December 2016, pp. 1996–2005.

Langer, Vijay, "Management of Major Limb Injuries," *Scientific World Journal*, Vol. 2014, January 2014.

LeBus, George F., and Cory Collinge, "Vascular Abnormalities as Assessed with CT Angiography in High-Energy Tibial Plafond Fractures," *Journal of Orthopaedic Trauma*, Vol. 22, No. 1, January 2008, pp. 16–22.

MacKenzie, Ellen J., Michael J. Bosse, Andrew N. Pollak, and Daniel J. Stinner, "The Major Extremity Trauma Research Consortium: An Overview," *Journal of Orthopaedic Trauma*, Vol. 31, April 2017, p. S1.

MacKenzie, E. J., M. J. Bosse, A. N. Pollak, L. X. Webb, M. F. Swiontkowski, J. F. Kellam, D. G. Smith, R. W. Sanders, A. L. Jones, A. J. Starr, M. P. McAndrew, B. M. Patterson, A. R. Burgess, and R. C. Castillo, "Long-Term Persistence of Disability Following Severe Lower-Limb Trauma: Results of a Seven-Year Follow-Up," *Journal of Bone and Joint Surgery*, Vol. 87, No. 8, August 2005, pp. 1801–1809.

MacKenzie, Ellen J., Renan C. Castillo, Alison Snow Jones, Michael J. Bosse, James F. Kellam, Andrew N. Pollak, Lawrence X. Webb, Marc F. Swiontkowski, Douglas G. Smith, Roy W. Sanders, Alan L. Jones, Adam J. Starr, Mark P. McAndrew, Brendan M. Patterson, and Andrew R. Burgess, "Health-Care Costs Associated with Amputation or Reconstruction of a Limb-Threatening Injury," *Journal of Bone & Joint Surgery*, Vol. 89, No. 8, August 2007, pp. 1685–1692.

Major Extremity Trauma Research Consortium (METRC), "Building a Clinical Research Network in Trauma Orthopaedics: The Major Extremity Trauma Research Consortium (METRC)," *Journal of Orthopaedic Trauma*, Vol. 30, No. 7, July 2016, pp. 353–361.

Mangan, Katharine I., Trevor D. Kingsbury, Brittney N. Mazzone, Marilynn P. Wyatt, and Kevin M. Kuhn, "Limb Salvage with Intrepid Dynamic Exoskeletal Orthosis Versus Transtibial Amputation: A Comparison of Functional Gait Outcomes," *Journal of Orthopaedic Trauma*, Vol. 30, No. 12, December 2016, pp. e390–e395.

Melcer, Ted, Jay Walker, Vibha Bhatnagar, Erin Richard, V. Franklin Sechriest II, and Michael Galarneau, "A Comparison of Four-Year Health Outcomes Following Combat Amputation and Limb Salvage," *PloS ONE*, Vol. 12, No. 1, January 2017.

Melcer, Ted, G. Jay Walker, V. Franklin Sechriest II, Michael Galarneau, Paula Konoske, and Jay Pyo, "Short-Term Physical and Mental Health Outcomes for Combat Amputee and Nonamputee Extremity Injury Patients," *Journal of Orthopaedic Trauma*, Vol. 27, No. 2, February 2013, pp. e31–e37.

Momoh, Adeyiza O., and Kevin C. Chung, "Measuring Outcomes in Lower Limb Surgery," *Clinics in Plastic Surgery*, Vol. 40, No. 2, April 2013, pp. 323–329.

Muscatelli, Stefano, Hayley Spurr, Nathan N. O'Hara, Lyndsay M. O'Hara, Sheila A. Sprague, and Gerard P. Slobogean, "Prevalence of Depression and Posttraumatic Stress Disorder After Acute Orthopaedic Trauma: A Systematic Review and Meta-Analysis," *Journal of Orthopaedic Trauma*, Vol. 31, No. 1, January 2017, pp. 47–55.

O'Toole, Robert V., Manjari Joshi, Anthony R. Carlini, Clinton K. Murray, Lauren E. Allen, Daniel O. Scharfstein, Joshua L. Gary, Michael J. Bosse, Renan C. Castillo, and Major Extremity Trauma Research Consortium (METRC), "Local Antibiotic Therapy to Reduce Infection After Operative Treatment of Fractures at High Risk of Infection: A Multicenter, Randomized, Controlled Trial (VANCO Study)," *Journal of Orthopaedic Trauma*, Vol. 31, Supplement 1, April 2017, pp. S18–S24.

Owens, Johnny G., James A. Blair, Jeanne C. Patzkowski, Ryan V. Blanck, Joseph R. Hsu, and the Skeletal Trauma Research Consortium (STReC), "Return to Running and Sports Participation After Limb Salvage," *Journal of Trauma: Injury, Infection, and Critical Care*, Vol. 71, No. 1, July 2011, pp. S120–S124.

Owens, Brett D., John F. Kragh, Jr., Joseph Macaitis, Steven J. Svoboda, and Joseph C. Wenke, "Characterization of Extremity Wounds in Operation Iraqi Freedom and Operation Enduring Freedom," *Journal of Orthopaedic Trauma*, Vol. 21, No. 4, April 2007, pp. 254–257.

Patzkowski, Jeanne C., Ryan V. Blanck, Johnny G. Owens, Jason M. Wilken, Kevin L. Kirk, Joseph C. Wenke, Joseph R. Hsu, and the Skeletal Trauma Research Consortium (STReC), "Comparative Effect of Orthosis Design on Functional Performance," *Journal of Bone and Joint Surgery*, Vol. 94, No. 6, March 2012, pp. 507–515.

Patzkowski, Jeanne C., Johnny G. Owens, Ryan V. Blanck, Kevin L. Kirk, and Joseph R. Hsu, "Deployment After Limb Salvage for High-Energy Lower-Extremity Trauma," *Journal of Trauma and Acute Care Surgery*, Vol. 73, No. 2, Supplement 1, August 2012, pp. S112–S115.

Penn-Barwell, J. G., R. W. Myatt, P. M. Bennett, I. D. Sargeant, on behalf of the Severe Lower Extremity Combat Trauma (SeLECT) Study Group, C. A. Fries, R. W. Myatt, J. M. Kendrew, M. J. Midwinter, R. F. Rickard, K. Porter, T. Rowlands, A. Mountain, M. Foster, S. Stapley, D. Mortiboy, and J. Bishop, "Medium-Term Outcomes Following Limb Salvage for Severe Open Tibia Fracture Are Similar to Trans-Tibial Amputation," *Injury*, Vol. 46, No. 2, February 2015, pp. 288–291.

Petfield, Joseph L., Garry T. Hayeck, David L. Kopperdahl, Leon J. Nesti, Tony M. Keaveny, Joseph R. Hsu, on behalf of the Skeletal Trauma Research Consortium (STReC), "Virtual Stress Testing of Fracture Stability in Soldiers with Severely Comminuted Tibial Fractures," *Journal of Orthopaedic Research*, Vol. 35, No. 4, April 2017, pp. 805–811.

Potter, Benjamin K., Robert G. Sheu, Daniel Stinner, John Fergason, Joseph R. Hsu, Kevin Kuhn, Johnny G. Owens, Jessica Rivera, Scott B. Shawen, Jason M. Wilken, Jennifer DeSanto, Yanjie Huang, Daniel O. Scharfstein, and Ellen J. MacKenzie, "Multisite Evaluation of a Custom Energy-Storing Carbon Fiber Orthosis for Patients with Residual Disability After Lower-Limb Trauma," *Journal of Bone and Joint Surgery*, Vol. 100, No. 20, October 2018, pp. 1781–1789.

Ramasamy, Arul, Stuart Harrisson, Irwin Lasrado, and Michael P. M. Stewart, "A Review of Casualties During the Iraqi Insurgency 2006—A British Field Hospital Experience," *Injury*, Vol. 40, No. 5, May 2009, pp. 493–497.

Rispoli, Damian M., and Ellen J. MacKenzie, "Orthopaedic Outcomes: Combat and Civilian Trauma Care," *Journal of the American Academy of Orthopaedic Surgeons*, Vol. 20, 2012, pp. S84–S87.

Rivera, Jessica C., Joseph C. Wenke, and Mary Jo Pugh, "Open Fracture Care During War: Opportunities for Research," *JB&JS Reviews*, Vol. 4, No. 10, October 2016.

Rush, Robert M., Jr., Edward D. Arrington, and Joseph R. Hsu, "Management of Complex Extremity Injuries: Tourniquets, Compartment Syndrome Detection, Fasciotomy, and Amputation Care," *Surgical Clinics of North America*, Vol. 92, No. 4, August 2012, pp. 987–1007.

Sabino, Jennifer M., Julia Slater, and Ian L. Valerio, "Plastic Surgery Challenges in War Wounded I: Flap-Based Extremity Reconstruction," *Advances in Wound Care*, Vol. 5, No. 9, September 2016, pp. 403–411.

Saddawi-Konefka, Daniel, Hyungjin Kim, and Kevin C. Chung, "A Systematic Review of Outcomes and Complications of Reconstruction and Amputation for Type IIIB and IIIC Fractures of the Tibia," *Plastic and Reconstructive Surgery*, Vol. 122, No. 6, December 2008, pp. 1796–1805.

Scalea, Joseph R., Robert Crawford, Stephanie Scurci, Jonathon Danquah, Rajabrata Sarkar, Joseph Kufera, James O'Connor, and Thomas M. Scalea, "Below-the-Knee Arterial Injury: The Type of Vessel May Be More Important Than the Number of Vessels Injured," *Journal of Trauma and Acute Care Surgery*, Vol. 77, No. 6, December 2014, pp. 920–925.

Scheulen, James J., and Andrew M. Munster, "The Parkland Formula in Patients with Burns and Inhalation Injury," *Journal of Trauma: Injury, Infection, and Critical Care*, Vol. 22, No. 10, October 1982, pp. 869–871.

Scott, Daniel J., J. Devin B. Watson, Thomas A. Heafner, Michael S. Clemens, Brandon W. Propper, and Zachary M. Arthurs, "Validation of the Short Musculoskeletal Function Assessment in Patients with Battlefield-Related Extremity Vascular Injuries," *Journal of Vascular Surgery*, Vol. 60, No. 6, December 2014, pp. 1620–1626.

Shaw, K. Aaron, Peter C. Johnson, David Williams, Steven D. Zumbrun, Richard Topolski, and Craig D. Cameron, "Chondrocyte Viability After a Simulated Blast Exposure," *Military Medicine*, Vol. 182, No. 7, July–August 2017, pp. e1941–e1947.

Sheean, Andrew J., Chad A. Krueger, and Joseph R. Hsu, "Return to Duty and Disability After Combat-Related Hindfoot Injury," *Journal of Orthopaedic Trauma*, Vol. 28, No. 11, November 2014, pp. e258–e262.

Sheean, Andrew J., David J. Tennent, Johnny G. Owens, Jason M. Wilken, Joseph R. Hsu, Daniel J. Stinner, and Skeletal Trauma Research Consortium (STReC), "Effect of Custom Orthosis and Rehabilitation Program on Outcomes Following Ankle and Subtalar Fusions," *Foot & Ankle International*, Vol. 37, No. 11, November 2016, pp. 1205–1210.

Shireman, Paula K., Todd E. Rasmussen, Carlos A. Jaramillo, and Mary Jo Pugh, "VA Vascular Injury Study (VAVIS): VA-DoD Extremity Injury Outcomes Collaboration," *BMC Surgery*, Vol. 15, No. 13, February 2015.

Siemionow, Maria, Adam Bobkiewicz, Joanna Cwykiel, Safak Uygur, and Wojciech Francuzik, "Epineural Sheath Jacket as a New Surgical Technique for Neuroma Prevention in the Rat Sciatic Nerve Model," *Annals of Plastic Surgery*, Vol. 79, No. 4, October 2017, pp. 377–384.

Soltanian, Hooman, Ryan M. Garcia, and Scott T. Hollenbeck, "Current Concepts in Lower Extremity Reconstruction," *Plastic and Reconstructive Surgery*, Vol. 136, No. 6, December 2015, pp. 815e–829e.

Spear, Abigail M., Emma M. Davies, Christopher Taylor, Rachel Whiting, Sara Macildowie, Emrys Kirkman, Mark Midwinter, and Sarah A. Watts, "Blast Wave Exposure to the Extremities Causes Endothelial Activation and Damage," *Shock*, Vol. 44, No. 5, November 2015, pp. 470–478.

Stinner, Daniel J., Joseph C. Wenke, James R. Ficke, Wade Gordon, James Toledano, Anthony R. Carlini, Daniel O. Scharfstein, Ellen J. MacKenzie, Michael J. Bosse, Joseph R. Hsu, and the Major Extremity Trauma Research Consortium (METRC), "Military and Civilian Collaboration: The Power of Numbers," *Military Medicine*, Vol. 182, Supplement 1, March 2017, pp. 10–17.

Teicher, Carrie, Nancy L. Foote, Ali M. K. Al Ani, Majd S. Alras, Sufyan I. Alqassab, Emmanuel Baron, Khalid Ahmed, Patrick Herard, and Rasheed M. Fakhri, "The Short Musculoskeletal Functional Assessment (SMFA) Score Amongst Surgical Patients with Reconstructive Lower Limb Injuries in War Wounded Civilians," *Injury*, Vol. 45, No. 12, December 2014, pp. 1996–2001.

Theodorakopoulou, Evgenia, Katrina A. Mason, Georgios Pafitanis, Ali M. Ghanem, Simon Myers, and Fortune C. Iwuagwu, "Free-Tissue Transfer for the Reconstruction of War-Related Extremity Injuries: A Systematic Review of Current Practice," *Military Medicine*, Vol. 181, No. 1, January 2016, pp. 27–34.

Tintle, Scott M., John J. Keeling, Scott B. Shawen, Jonathan A. Forsberg, and Benjamin K. Potter, "Traumatic and Trauma-Related Amputations: Part I: General Principles and Lower-Extremity Amputations," *Journal of Bone and Joint Surgery*, Vol. 92, No. 17, December 2010, pp. 2852–2868.

Tunali, O., Y. Saglam, H. I. Balci, A. Kochai, N. A. Sahbaz, O. A. Sayin, and O. Yazicioglu, "Gustilo Type IIIC Open Tibia Fractures with Vascular Repair: Minimum 2-Year Follow-Up," *European Journal of Trauma and Emergency Surgery*, Vol. 43, No. 4, August 2017, pp. 505–512.

U.S. Department of Defense Blast Injury Research Program Coordinating Office, *Minimizing the Impact of Wound Infections Following Blast-Related Injuries: 2016 State-of-the-Science Meeting Report Proceedings, Key Findings, and Expert Panel Recommendations*, Fort Detrick, Md., 2016a. As of April 6, 2020: https://blastinjuryresearch.amedd.army.mil/assets/docs/sos/ meeting_proceedings/2016_SoS_Meeting_Proceedings.pdf

———, *Minimizing the Impact of Wound Infections Following Blast-Related Injuries: Literature Review*, Fort Detrick, Md., 2016b. As of April 6, 2020: https://blastinjuryresearch.amedd.army.mil/assets/docs/sos/lit_reviews/ 2016_SoS_Literature_Review.pdf

Van der Merwe, Lana, Franz Birkholtz, Kevin Tetsworth, and Erik Hohmann, "Functional and Psychological Outcomes of Delayed Lower Limb Amputation Following Failed Lower Limb Reconstruction," *Injury*, Vol. 47, No. 8, August 2016, pp. 1756–1760.

Vincent, Heather K., MaryBeth Horodyski, Kevin R. Vincent, Sonya T. Brisbane, and Kalia K. Sadasivan, "Psychological Distress After Orthopedic Trauma: Prevalence in Patients and Implications for Rehabilitation," *PM&R*, Vol. 7, No. 9, September 2015, pp. 978–989.

Wallum, Timothy E., Heather C. Yun, Elizabeth A. Rini, Kristina Carter, Charles H. Guymon, Kevin S. Akers, Stuart D. Tyner, Christopher E. White, and Clinton K. Murray, "Pathogens Present in Acute Mangled Extremities from Afghanistan and Subsequent Pathogen Recovery," *Military Medicine*, Vol. 180, No. 1, January 2015, pp. 97–103.

Ward, Catherine L., Lisa Ji, and Benjamin T. Corona, "An Autologous Muscle Tissue Expansion Approach for the Treatment of Volumetric Muscle Loss," *Bioresearch Open Access*, Vol. 4, No. 1, March 2015, pp. 198–208.

Wegener, Stephen T., Renan C. Castillo, Sara E. Heins, Anna N. Bradford, Mary Zadnik Newell, Andrew Pollak, and Ellen J. MacKenzie, "The Development and Validation of the Readiness to Engage in Self-Management After Acute Traumatic Injury Questionnaire," *Rehabilitation Psychology*, Vol. 59, No. 2, May 2014, pp. 203–210.

Wegener, Stephen T., Andrew N. Pollak, Katherine P. Frey, Robert A. Hymes, Kristin R. Archer, Clifford B. Jones, Rachel B. Seymour, Robert V. O'Toole, Renan C. Castillo, Yanjie Huang, Daniel O. Scharfstein, Ellen J. MacKenzie, and METRC, "The Trauma Collaborative Care Study (TCCS)," *Journal of Orthopaedic Trauma*, Vol. 31, No. 4, April 2017, pp. S78–S87.

Whitehead, Jennifer M. Aldridge, Elizabeth Russell Esposito, and Jason M. Wilken, "Stair Ascent and Descent Biomechanical Adaptations While Using a Custom Ankle–Foot Orthosis," *Journal of Biomechanics*, Vol. 49, No. 13, September 2016, pp. 2899–2908.

Wilken, Jason M., Catherine W. Roy, Scott W. Shaffer, Jeanne C. Patzkowski, Ryan V. Blanck, Johnny G. Owens, and Joseph R. Hsu, "Physical Performance Limitations After Severe Lower Extremity Trauma in Military Service Members," *Journal of Orthopaedic Trauma*, Vol. 32, No. 4, April 2018, pp. 183–189.

Williams, Gavin, Bridget Hill, and Michelle Kahn, "The Concurrent Validity and Responsiveness of the High-Level Mobility Assessment Tool for Mobility Limitations in People with Multitrauma Orthopedic Injuries," *PM&R*, Vol. 6, No. 3, March 2014, pp. 235–240.

Young-McCaughan, Stacey, Mona O. Bingham, Catherine A. Vriend, Alice W. Inman, Kathryn M. Gaylord, and Christine Miaskowski, "The Impact of Symptom Burden on the Health Status of Service Members with Extremity Trauma," *Nursing Outlook*, Vol. 65, No. 5, September–October 2017, pp. S61–S70.